The Multiple Sclerosis Cookbook

By, Laura Hizak

Introduction

Thank you for purchasing this cookbook to benefit Multiple Sclerosis.

Allow me to introduce myself, my name is Laura. I have relapsing remitting multiple sclerosis and was diagnosed in 2006. I quickly realized that I had to do more to combat this disease, as until there is a cure medication alone is not enough. I discovered that a diet low in saturated fats was highly recommended for the benefit of multiple sclerosis. I adjusted my diet accordingly and have been living symptom free ever since.

First I would like to begin by telling you that I am not a professional chef. All of the following recipes were made in my basic kitchen at home. My family enjoyed eating the dishes especially the desserts, after I photographed them to share with you.

It is my mission to share the huge benefits that simply eating better can have for people with multiple sclerosis. I went back to school and studied holistic nutrition and began my journey to share my success with others.

The recipes in this book are my daily go to ones. They are all easy, inexpensive and quick.

As people living with multiple sclerosis it is important to take an active approach to helping ourselves to feel as good as possible. Eating better can be a huge factor in our health and in turn our happiness.

Research shows that a diet low in saturated fats can be of huge benefit to us. Many of the recipes in this book are without meat or dairy. I have however included some chicken recipes that you can try making with an alternative product, such as a soy based product. I recommend using this book to slowly introduce yourself to meat free cooking. Try making the switch from dairy milk to an alternative such as soy, almond, cashew, oat or rice milk.

As for the 'yummy treats' section be aware that the recipes containing chocolate contain saturated fat and should therefore be consumed in extreme moderation.

There are so many alternatives available for following a healthy low saturated fat diet. My hope is that by using the simple recipes in this book that you can slowly make the necessary changes to better your health.

The recipes in this book have allowed me to remain symptom & progression free for over 10 years & counting. These small dietary changes plus some simple lifestyle changes have allowed me to continue being an active mother to my two boys. They have also allowed me to maintain my high activity levels and most importantly they have NOT allowed multiple sclerosis to negatively impact my life whatsoever.

"Let food be thy medicine and medicine be thy food."
Hippocrates.

*In this book all oven temperatures are referring to a Fan Oven, please adjust accordingly

Table of Contents

Sauces

Fat Free Béchamel

500ml fat free milk \ Soy milk
2 heaped tbsp corn flour
1tsp nutmeg
Pinch of black pepper

- Add all ingredients to a medium sized pot, set to a low temperature
- Whisking constantly allow the sauce to thicken

- Perfect for lasagna, follow the Bolognese recipe in this book, layer lasagna pasta sheets with the Bolognese & this béchamel sauce, then bake covered with foil, in a pre-heated fan oven at 180 for 35 minutes

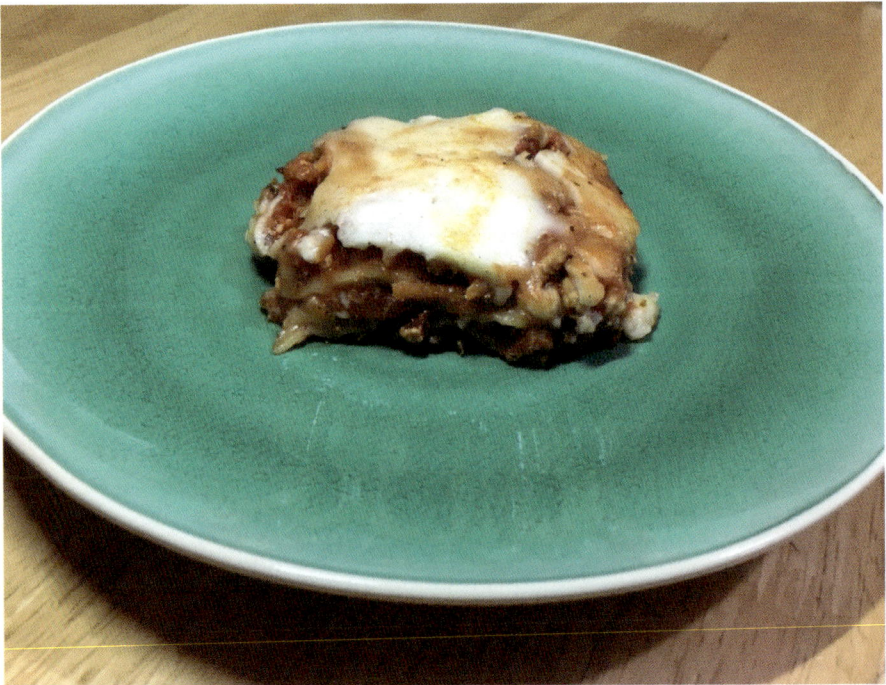

Pizza or Pasta Sauce

This sauce is perfect for pizza, Bolognese or just simply mixed with plain pasta.

250g cherry tomatoes
2 tbsp tomato purée
1 tsp garlic powder
Salt & Pepper
1 tin of chopped tomatoes
Big glug of red wine
2 tbsp oregano
Pinch of sugar

- Put everything in a large pot, bring to a boil then simmer for 10-15 minutes, blend with a hand blender,
- That's it, finished!

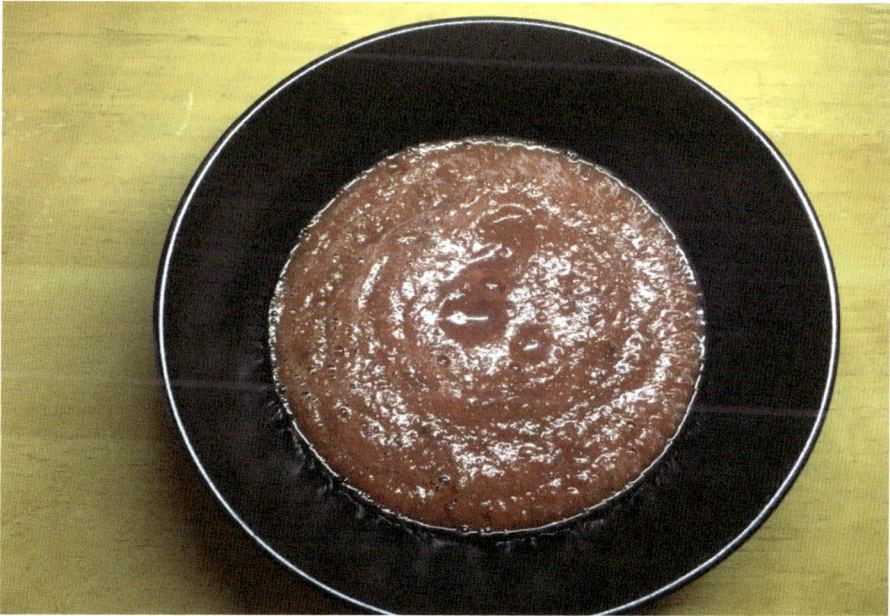

Soups

Carrot & Coriander Soup

2 tbsp olive oil

1 medium onion, chopped

1 celery stalk, chopped

1 ltr vegetable stock

2-3 leafy celery stalks, chopped

2 small potatoes, chopped

3 tsp ground coriander

1lb carrots, chopped

- Heat the olive oil in a large pot add onion, celery & potatoes, cook on a medium heat stirring frequently until the potatoes begin to soften.

- Add in the carrots & leave to soften for roughly 10 minutes, stirring frequently

- Add in the stock leave for another 10 minutes

- In a separate frying pan dry fry the ground coriander until you can smell it strongly add in the chopped leafy celery stalks and mix well

- Add the fried coriander mixture to the soup

- Use a hand blender to purée the soup

- Serve with fresh soda bread

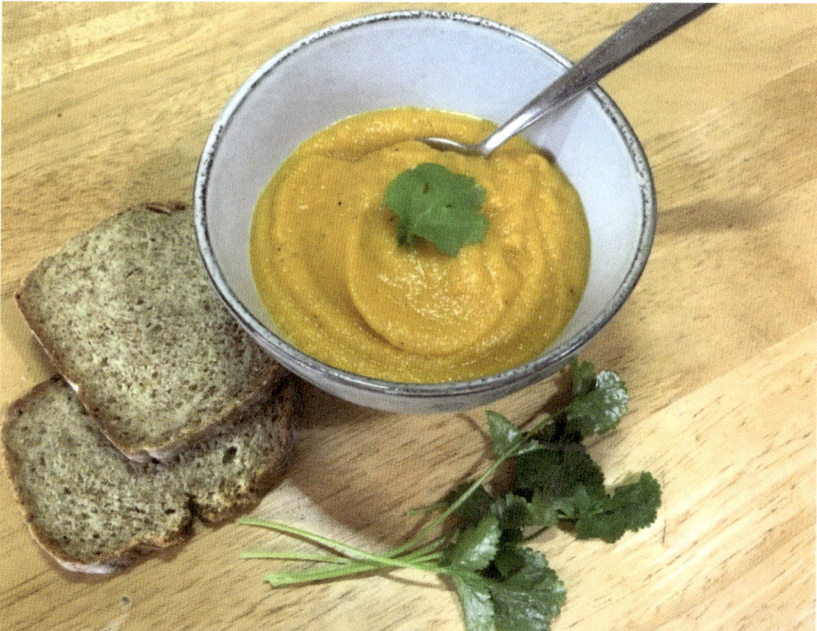

Chicken Noodle Soup

900ml chicken stock

2 chicken breasts

1tsp root ginger, grated

2 garlic cloves, crushed

2 tbsp sweet corn

3 scallions, sliced

 3 button mushrooms

2 tbsp soy sauce

50g noodles of your choice

- Place the raw chicken breasts in a large pot with the stock, ginger and garlic & bring to a boil, then simmer for 20 minutes
- Remove the chicken from the pot onto a chopping board and use two forks to tear the chicken breasts into shreds
- Add the noodles into the stock mixture and cook as per packet instructions add the sweet corn, mushrooms, soy sauce and the shredded chicken back into the stock
- Serve sprinkled with chopped scallions

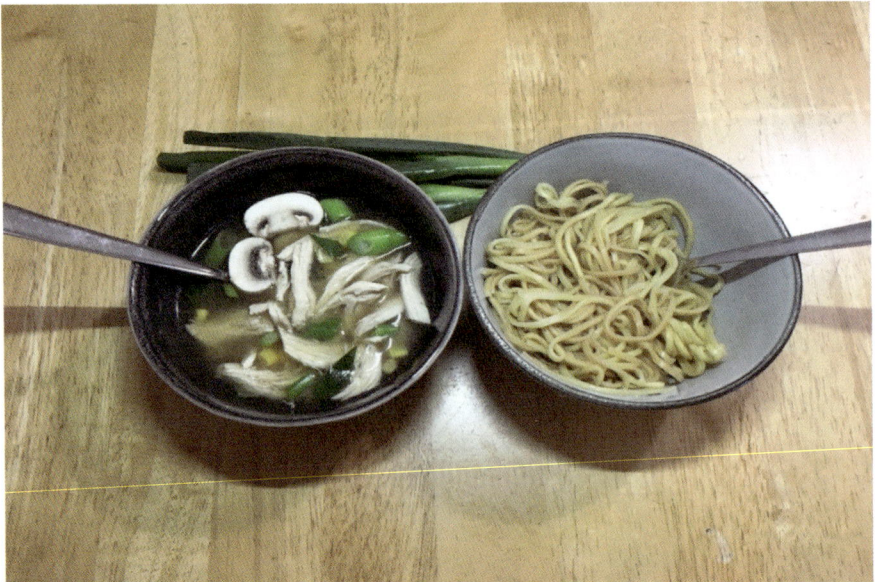

Leek and Potato Soup

• •

500g fresh leeks, washed & chopped
500g potatoes, peeled & chopped
1 celery stalk, chopped

3 tbsp olive oil

1 medium onion, chopped
1.5 ltr chicken or vegetable stock
1 bay leaf

Salt & Pepper

- Heat the olive oil in a large pot add in all veg including potatoes, cook over a medium heat roughly 10-15 minutes stirring frequently to prevent sticking
- Add the stock & bay leaf
- Bring to a boil then reduce heat and simmer until all potatoes & veg are cooked
- Remove bay leaf, then blend using a hand blender
- Season to preferred taste
- Serve with fresh soda bread

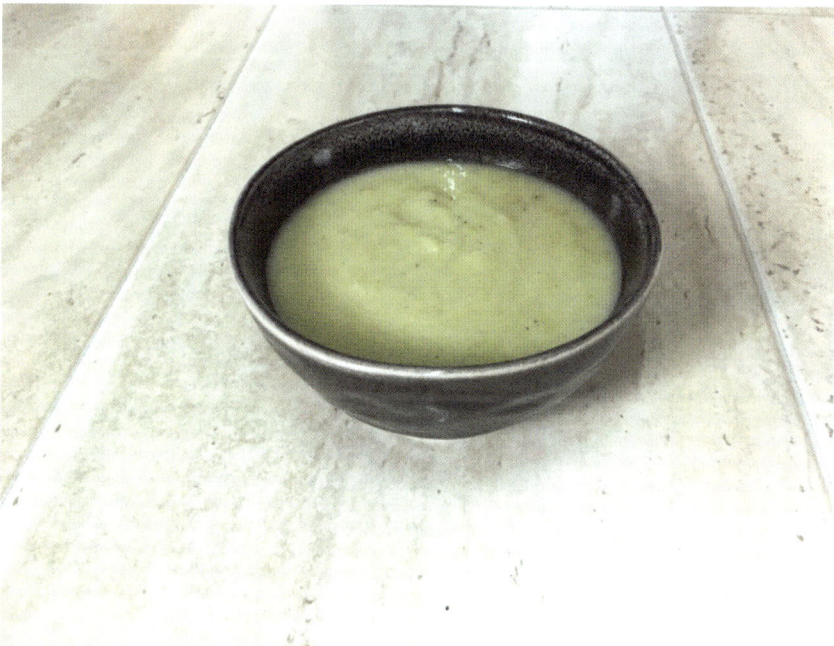

Chickpea and Turkey Bacon Soup

Vegeta is the ultimate flavor enhancer, originally produced in Croatia.

1 tbsp olive oil

1 medium onion, grated

6 slices turkey bacon, chopped

2 garlic cloves, crushed

1.5 ltr water

1 celery stalk chopped

1 tbsp chopped celery leaf

1 can chickpeas, rinsed

2 tbsp tomato purée

2 bay leaves

200g small pasta shells

1 tsp Vegeta - available in most European food stores

- Heat the olive oil in a large pot, add the onion and bacon with a little of the water
- Add vegeta, bay leaves, celery leaves and celery, continue cooking on a medium heat roughly 10 minutes
- Meanwhile cook the pasta as per packet instructions, once cooked rinse with boiled water and leave to the side
- Cover the bacon mixture with the rest of the water, add the chickpeas and tomato purée, bring to a boil then simmer for 5-10 minutes
- Serve in large bowls adding the pasta to each bowl separately

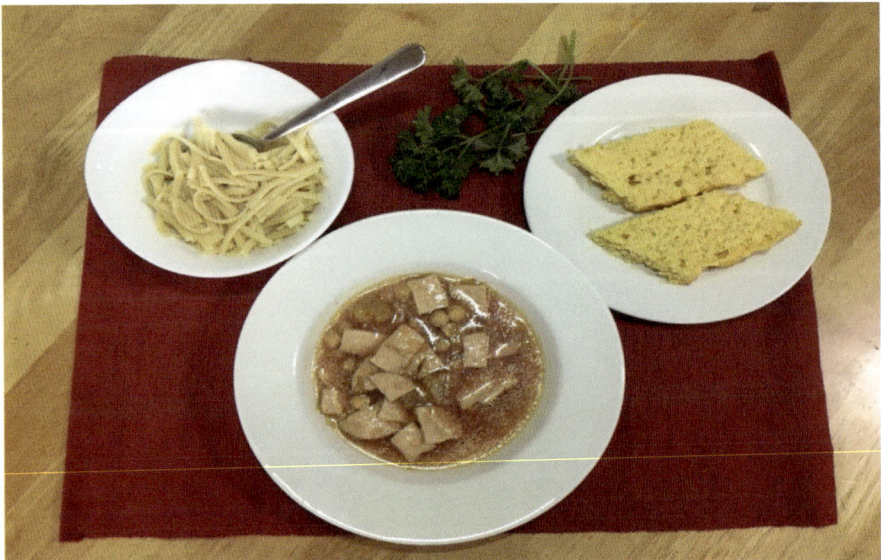

Sides

Colcannon

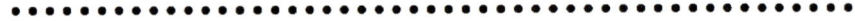

4 large potatoes, peeled
200g green cabbage, shredded
1/4 tsp garlic powder
200ml fat free milk\soy milk
20ml olive oil
Salt

- Boil the potatoes in salted water until softened
- In a separate pot boil the cabbage in salted water until it becomes soft
- Once the potatoes have softened, drain & then mash using a potato masher, adding the olive oil, milk, garlic & salt to taste.
- Use a hand blender to purée the potatoes
- Drain the cabbage then add it to the potato purée & mix well

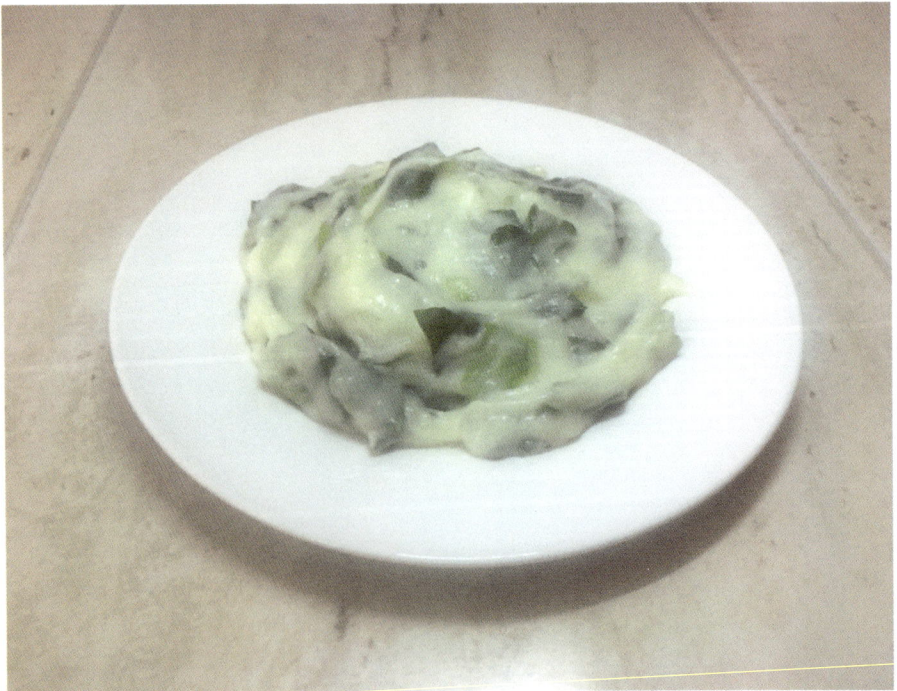

Chips / French Fries

● ●

This recipe is perfect with sweet potato too! Cooking for Multiple Sclerosis is all about low saturated fat so if you've got a 'chip-pan' or deep fat fryer please do yourself a favor and get rid of it, anything that can be cooked in a deep fat fryer can be done in the oven with half the fat!

4 large potatoes, peeled & cut into shape
2-3 tbsp olive oil
1 tsp garlic powder
2 tsp paprika
Salt and Pepper
1 large zip lock bag

- Place the cut potatoes into the Zip lock bag
- Add the remaining ingredients, seal the bag and shake to coat all the potatoes
- Pour out onto a large baking tray and bake in the center of a preheated oven on a medium heat until cooked through

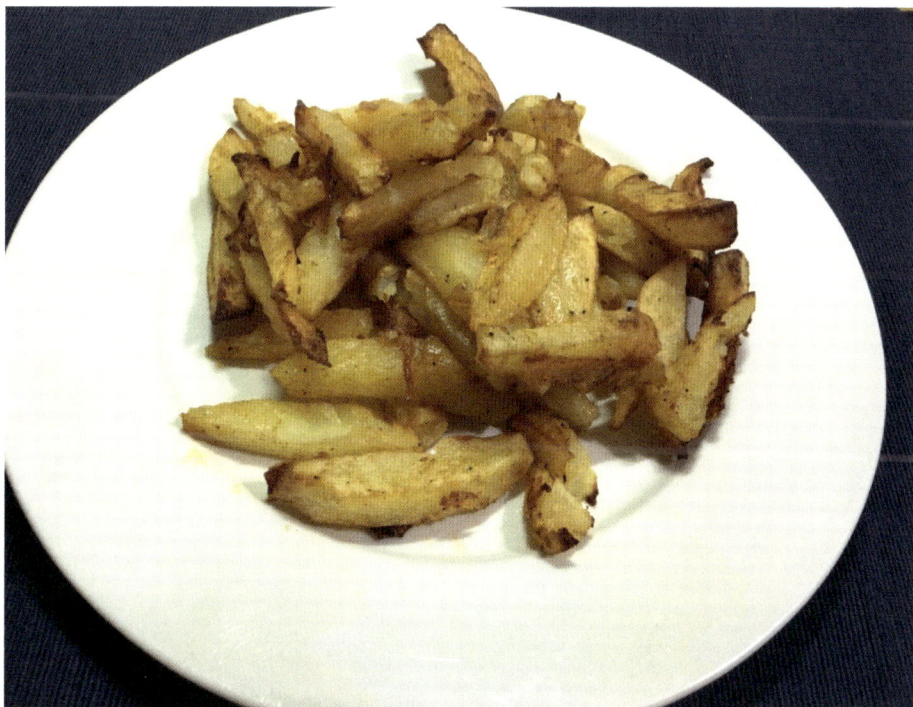

Fancy Garlic Bread

· ·

This is the most basic, simple recipe but sometimes it's the simple things that are the best!

1 French baguette

5-6 cherry tomatoes, roughly chopped

3 garlic cloves, crushed

4 tbsp olive oil

1 tbsp Italian herbs

- In a blender combine all ingredients for topping
- Carefully slice the baguette in slices but not completely through
- Place the baguette on a lined baking sheet
- Use a teaspoon to spoon the mixture in between each slice
- Bake in the oven on a medium heat until the bread is warm and crispy

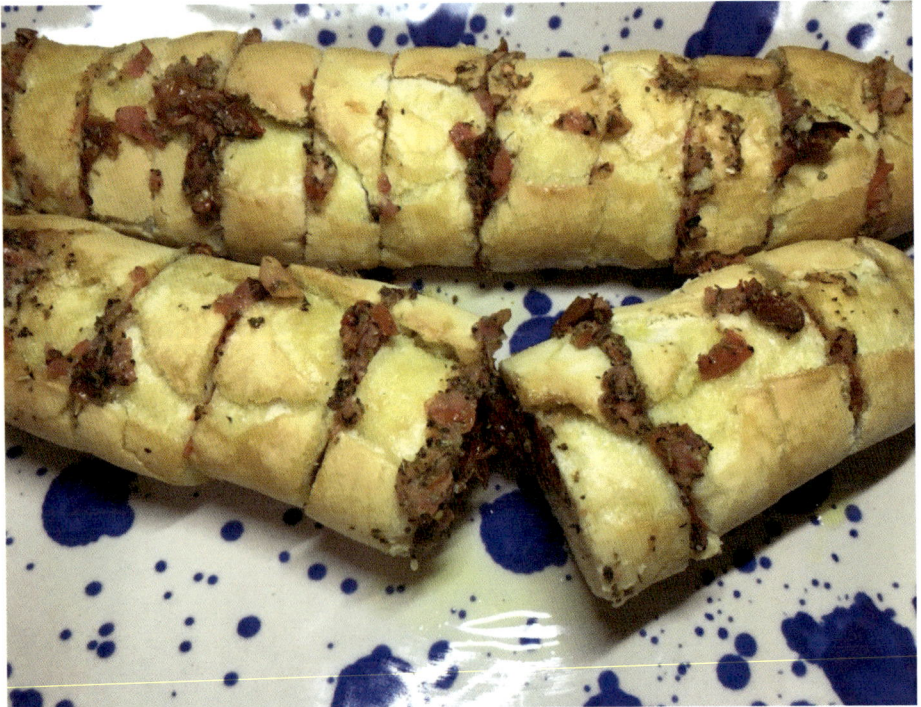

Cornbread

350g self raising flour
170g yellow corn flour
2tsp baking powder
1/2 tsp salt
75ml rapeseed oil
1 egg, beaten
300ml non fat milk

- In a large mixing bowl, mix all of the dry ingredients add in all of the wet ones and mix well

- Preheat the oven to 170 degrees

- Pour the mixture into a greased & lined baking tin

- Bake in the centre of the oven for 25-30 minutes, until a wooden skewer inserted into the middle comes out clean

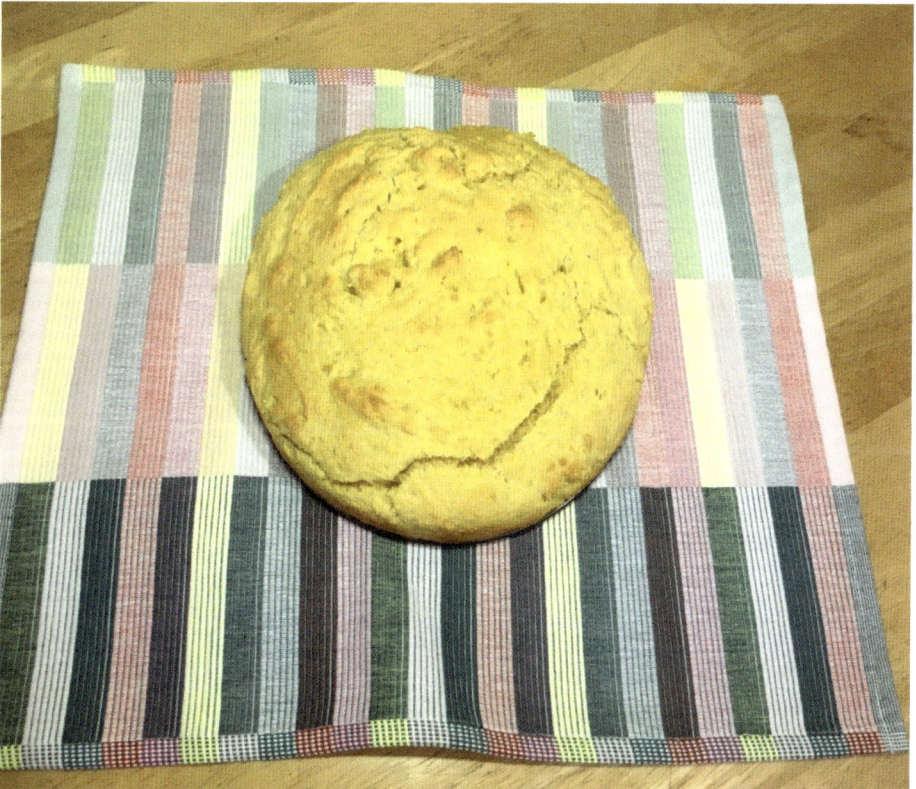

Gnocchi

100g mashed potatoes
25g plain flour
1 egg, beaten
Salt & Pepper

- In a large bowl mix all ingredients together to form a stiff dough add more flour if necessary
- Sprinkle a work surface with flour & roll the gnocchi dough out into a large sausage shape, use a knife to cut it into 1 inch (roughly) pieces, then roll between the palms of your hands to form round shapes
- Bring a large pan of salted water to the boil, drop the gnocchi directly into the boiling water in small batches
- Cook until the gnocchi are floating plus 2 minutes
- Serve immediately

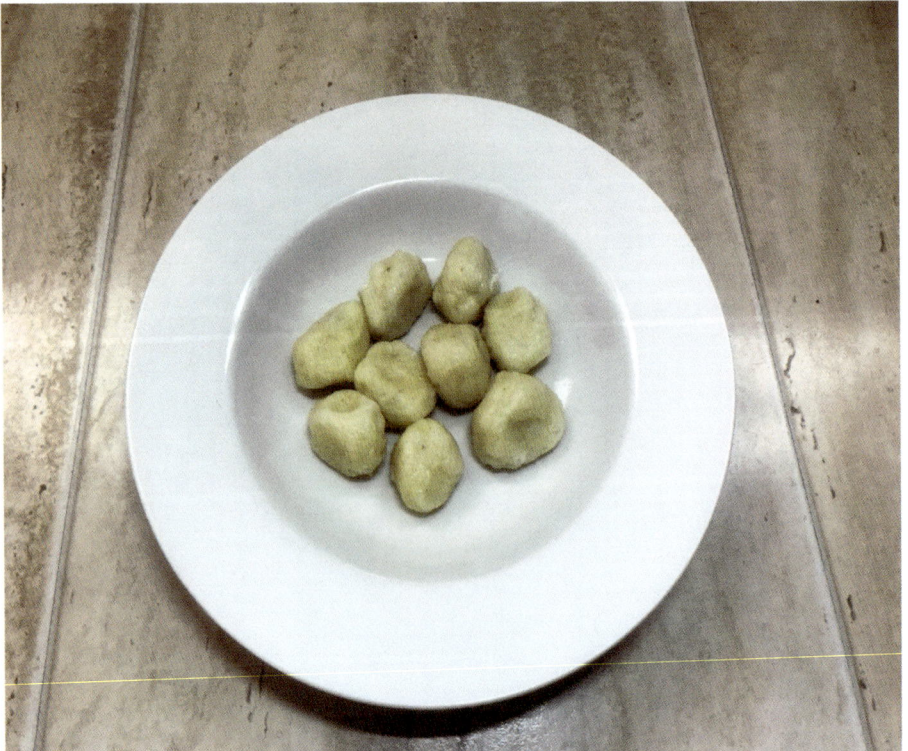

Mains

Bolognese

2-3tbsp olive oil

1 large carrot, grated

1 medium onion, grated

1 celery stalk, grated

400g turkey mince or 1/2 bag soy mince

4-6 button mushrooms, chopped

Salt & Pepper

1 tin chopped tomatoes

3 tbsp tomato purée

3tsp oregano

2 tsp basil

1/2 tsp garlic powder

pinch brown sugar

100ml red wine

- Add the carrot, onion, celery & olive oil to a large pot, sweat the vegetables
- Add the turkey mince or soy mince directly from the freezer & continue cooking until it is cooked through then add the mushrooms
- Mix well & allow to cook for 5-10 minutes
- Add the tomato puree & tinned tomatoes, stirring well then add the herbs, garlic, salt, pepper, bay leaves & wine
- Mix well then allow the Bolognese to come to a boil then cover & simmer 15- 20 minutes
- Remove bay leaves before serving

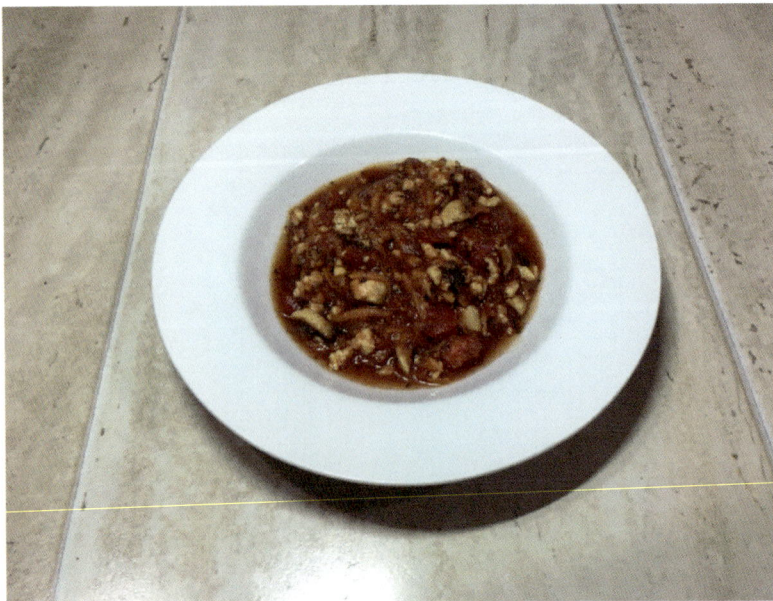

Honey Cashew Nut Chicken

1 tbsp olive oil

1/2 tsp chili flakes

1 large handful of cashew nuts

4 Chicken breasts, diced

For the Sauce

2 cloves garlic, crushed

1 inch piece ginger, grated

75ml runny honey

50ml light soy sauce

1 tbsp white wine vinegar

1-2 tbsp corn flour

200ml water

2 scallions, sliced

- Mix all sauce ingredients and leave to sit
- Meanwhile in a large frying pan add the olive oil, cashew nuts and chili flakes, gently fry until lightly browned
- Remove the nuts from the pan & leave to sit on a sheet of kitchen paper
- In the same pan fry the diced chicken breasts or soy chicken pieces until cooked through
- Pour the sauce over the cooked chicken & allow to thicken while mixing
- Once the sauce has thickened add in the cashew nuts
- Serve with boiled rice

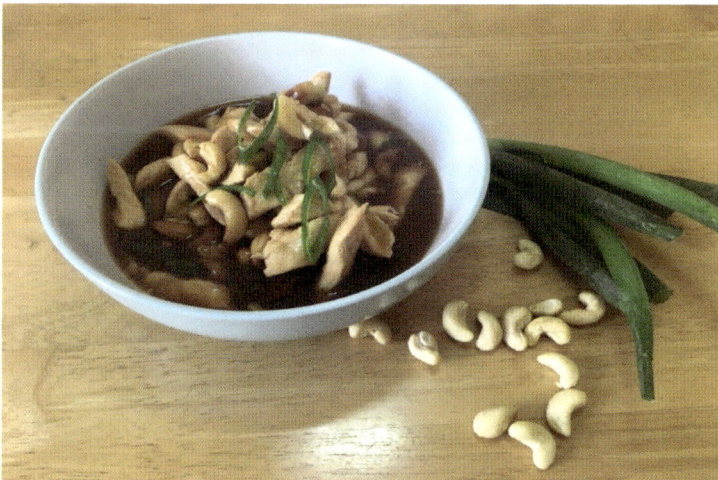

Mushroom Burgers

4 large mushrooms or 6-8 chopped small mushrooms
2 tbsp olive oil
2 tbsp balsamic vinegar
1 tsp oregano
1 tsp basil
2 garlic cloves, crushed
To Serve -
4 brioche burger buns
1 avocado
Tomato relish
Rocket leaves

- Mix the olive oil, vinegar, garlic, herbs, salt and pepper
- Either mix the chopped mushrooms directly into the vinegar mix or place the large mushrooms onto a tin foil coated baking sheet and coat both sides of the mushrooms with the mixture.
- Allow to marinade for 10-15 minutes
- If using small chopped mushrooms, fry them on a frying pan until cooked to your preference, alternatively place the large mushrooms under a hot grill & grill 3-5 minutes per side
- Lightly toast the brioche buns, mash the avocado and stack the mushroom burgers with the avocado, relish, rocket salad & mushrooms

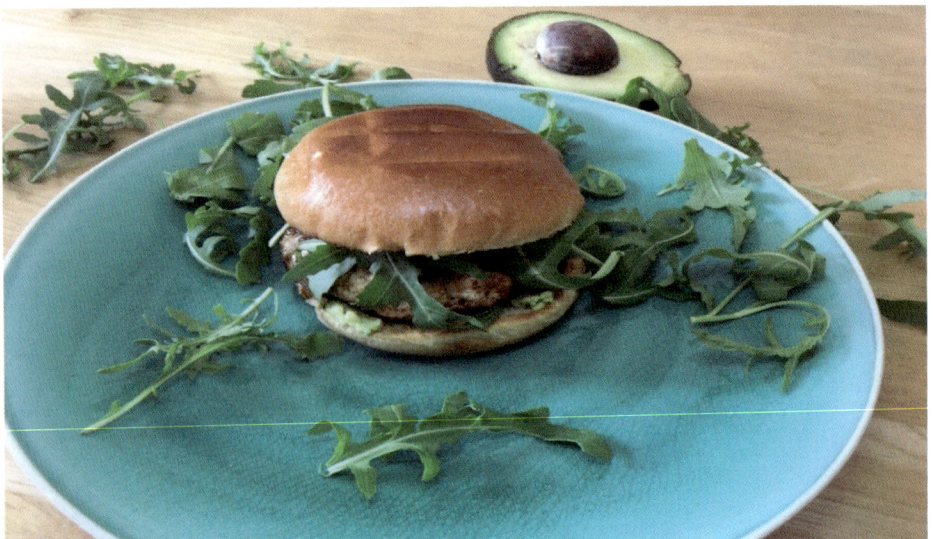

Pizza Dough

450ml water
1 Sachet yeast
1 tbsp brown sugar
750kg pizza flour + extra for rolling & prep
1 tsp salt
200ml sunflower oil

- Heat the water to between 33-39 degrees, use a thermometer to be precise it makes for much better dough
- Add sugar & allow to dissolve while maintaining the temperature at all times
- Add the sachet of yeast to the water and leave 10-15 minutes to foam & rise, monitor the temp during this time
- In a large metal bowl add the flour & salt, mix well
- Make a well in the center and once the yeast mixture has risen add it to the flour add the sunflower oil then mix well
- Pour the mixture out onto a wooden surface and knead well, using extra flour if necessary.
- Wash the metal bowl then brush with oil
- Place the dough into the greased bowl and cover with cling film, leave in a warm place to rise.
- Once risen take large handfuls to roll out into pizzas

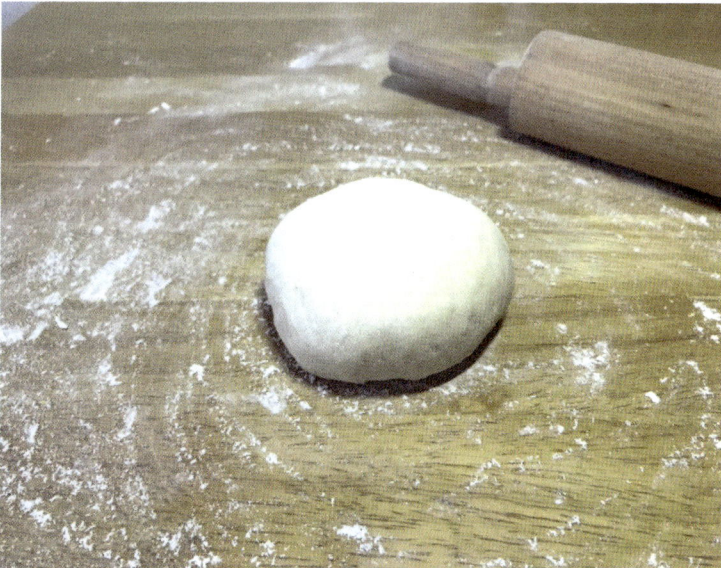

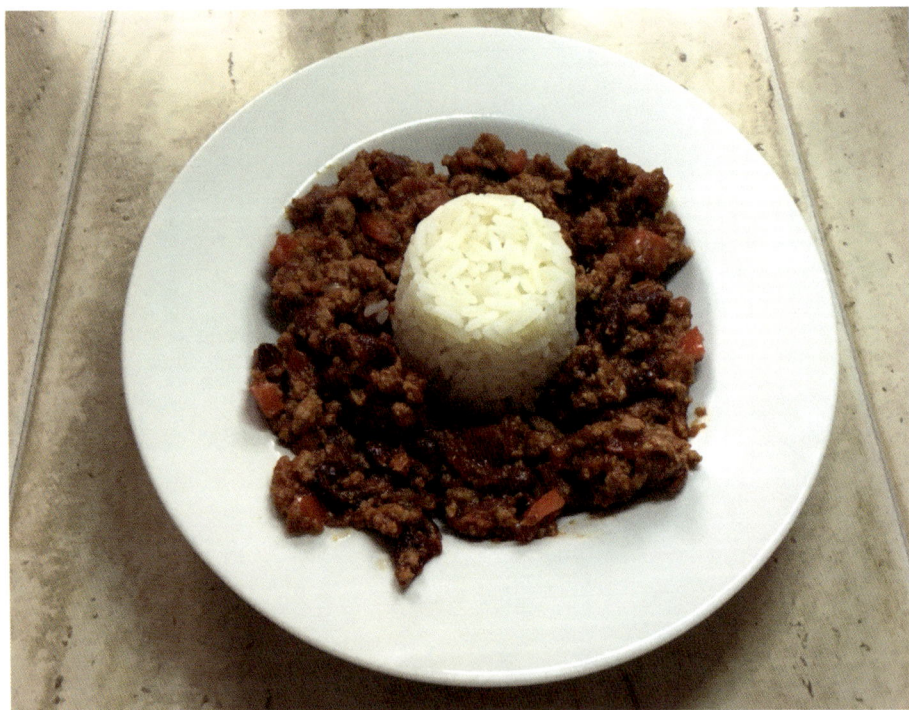

Chili

- -

1 garlic clove, crushed

1 tsp chili powder

1 tsp cumin

1 tsp paprika

2 stock cubes

1/2 tsp marjoram

1 tin chopped tomatoes

1 tbsp olive oil

1 large onion, grated

1 red pepper, grated

2 tbsp tomato purée

1 tin kidney beans, drained & rinsed

1 packet soy mince \ 4 chicken breasts chopped

- If using frozen soy mince first break it up before opening the packet
- Mix all spices with the meat/soy meat & allow to sit for at least 30 minutes, overnight if possible
- In a large pot sweat the onion, pepper and garlic
- Add the meat and stir until cooked through
- Add the water, stock cube, tinned tomatoes, tomato purée, salt & pepper
- Bring to a boil, then leave to simmer stirring occasionally until the water has been absorbed
- Add the kidney beans to the chili
- Bring to a boil again then remove the chili from the heat & allow it to sit for 30 minutes
- Reheat & serve with rice
- Prefect as a taco filling

3 Way Tomato, Spinach & Mushroom Pasta

4 servings of pasta

1 tbsp olive oil
3 garlic cloves, crushed
250g button mushrooms, diced
250g cherry tomatoes, halved
6 sun-dried tomatoes
3 tbsp tomato purée
3 tbsp soy sauce
1 tsp paprika
2 handfuls of fresh baby leaf spinach

- Cook the pasta as per pack instructions
- Fry the garlic with a sprinkle of salt & pepper in the olive oil, add the mushrooms and cherry tomatoes, fry for 5-7 minutes.
- Add the sun-dried tomatoes and continue to cook 2-3 minutes, add the chili flakes, tomato purée, soy sauce and paprika to the mushroom mix
- Lastly add the fresh spinach and allow to wilt, mix with the cooked pasta
- Serve with sea salt

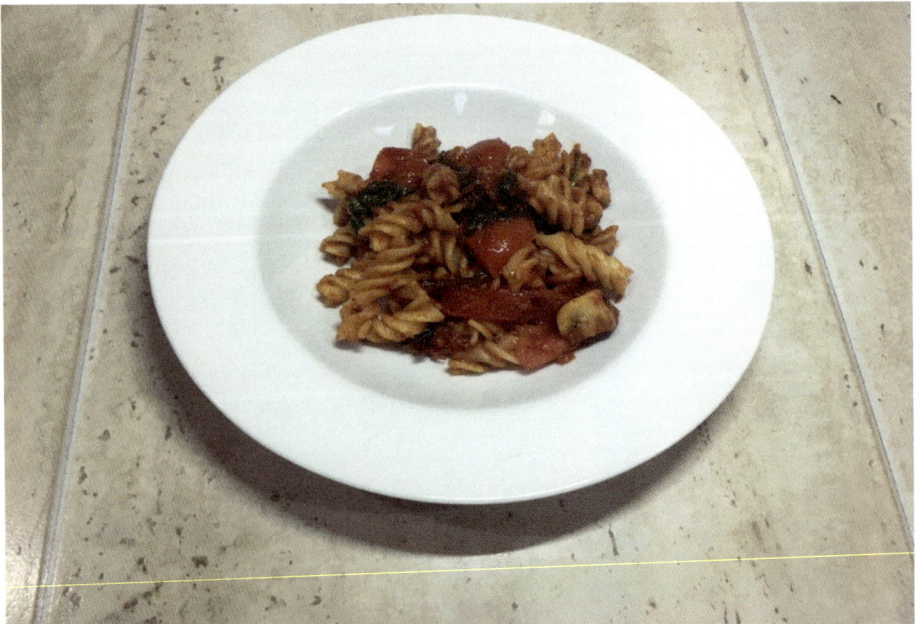

Cod Cakes

500g fresh cod, boned & skinned
75g breadcrumbs
100ml water
1 onion, grated
1 egg
2-3 tbsp sunflower oil
Salt & Pepper

- Mix the breadcrumbs with the water & leave to soak
- Place the cod in a food processor with the onion & blend
- Add the blended fish to the breadcrumbs mixture add in the egg, salt & pepper & mix well
- Heat the oil on a large pan & using wet hands shape the cod mixture into small patties
- Fry 5-6 minutes per side or until cooked through

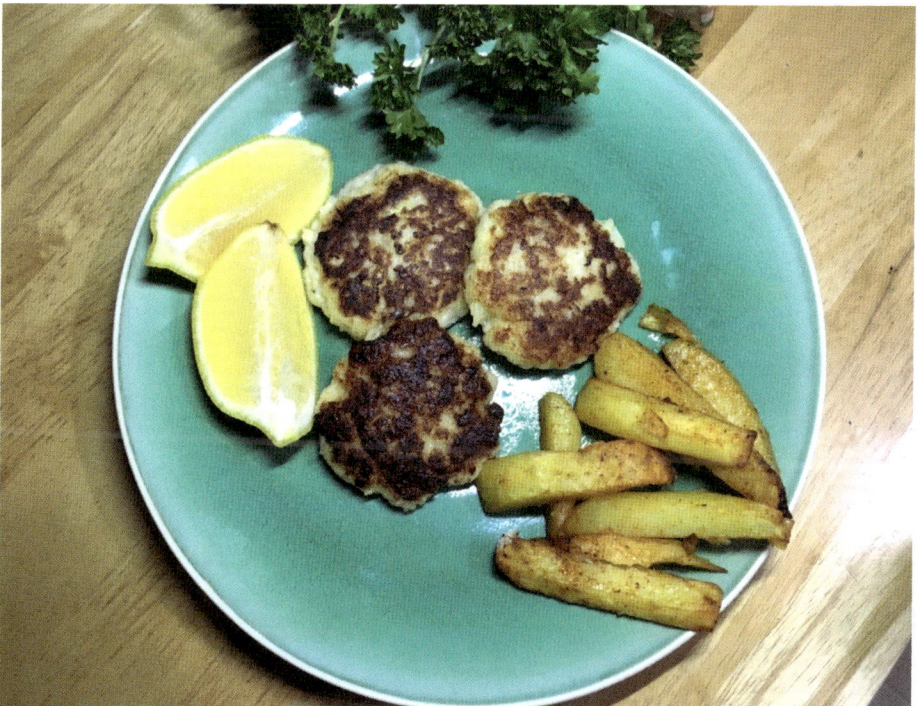

Honey Mustard Schnitzels

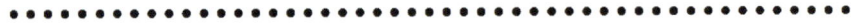

4 chicken breasts, pounded flat
3 tbsp mustard
3 tbsp runny honey
50g breadcrumbs

- Place the chicken breasts between two sheets of cling film & pound flat using a mallet
- In a small bowl mix the honey & mustard, place the breadcrumbs in a large deep flat plate
- Coat the chicken in the mustard & honey mixture then coat with the breadcrumbs
- Place the coated chicken on a grease proof lined baking tray & bake in a pre-heated oven on a medium heat until cooked through
- This can be made with frozen soy 'chicken' too, simply add the soy chicken to a large pan with a tbsp oil add the honey mustard mixture & 2tbsp breadcrumbs, top with chopped scallions.

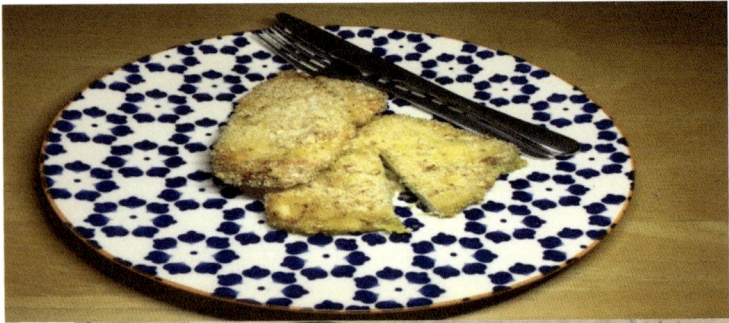

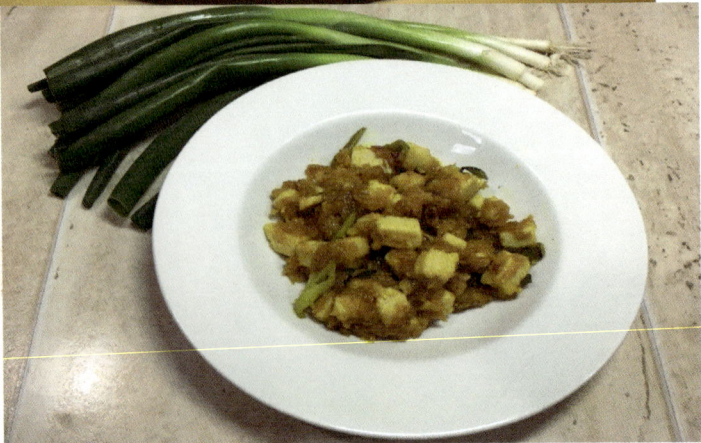

Soy mince & Potato Curry

- -

450g soy mince

300g potatoes, cubed

2 medium onions, grated

1 tsp fresh ginger, grated

2 garlic cloves, crushed

1 tsp coriander

1 tsp turmeric

1 tsp salt

1 tsp chili powder

1 tsp garam masala

2-3 fresh tomatoes, chopped

2 tbsp plain soy yogurt

- Fry the onions in a splash of oil add in the frozen soy mince, break it up
with a spatula, add in the garlic, ginger and cook until the mince is thawed
- Add in all spices & 3-4 tbsp water, cook for 2minutes
- Add in the tomatoes & yogurt, cook for a further 10 minutes on a low
heat
- Add potatoes mix well, add 1 cup of water & cook until potatoes have
softened, stir frequently
- Serve with rice or folded between a sheet of savory dough to make pies (see
  pie crust recipe in yummy treats section) & baked at 180degrees 45-50 mins

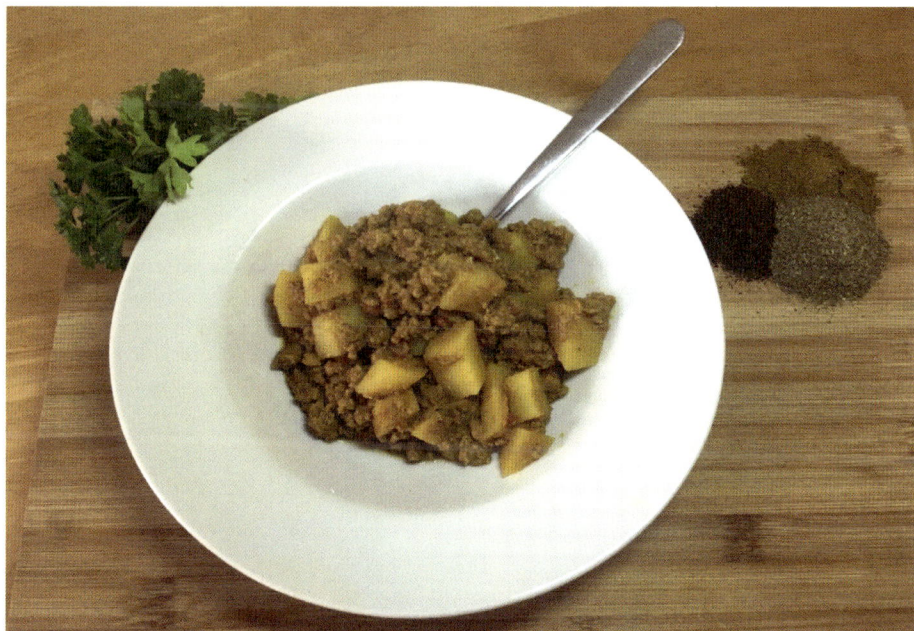

Spinach Gnocchi

• •

500g gnocchi
2 garlic cloves, crushed
150g fresh baby leaf spinach
2 tbsp frozen peas
1 tbsp rapeseed oil
1/4 tsp chili flakes
250ml reduced fat cream \ soy cream

- Cook the gnocchi as per recipe in this book, alternatively cook as per pack instructions
- In a large pan heat the oil, fry garlic & chili add in spinach & allow to wilt
- Add in the peas & cream, stir well
- Add the gnocchi
- Serve immediately with sea salt, parmesan & if desired Tabasco

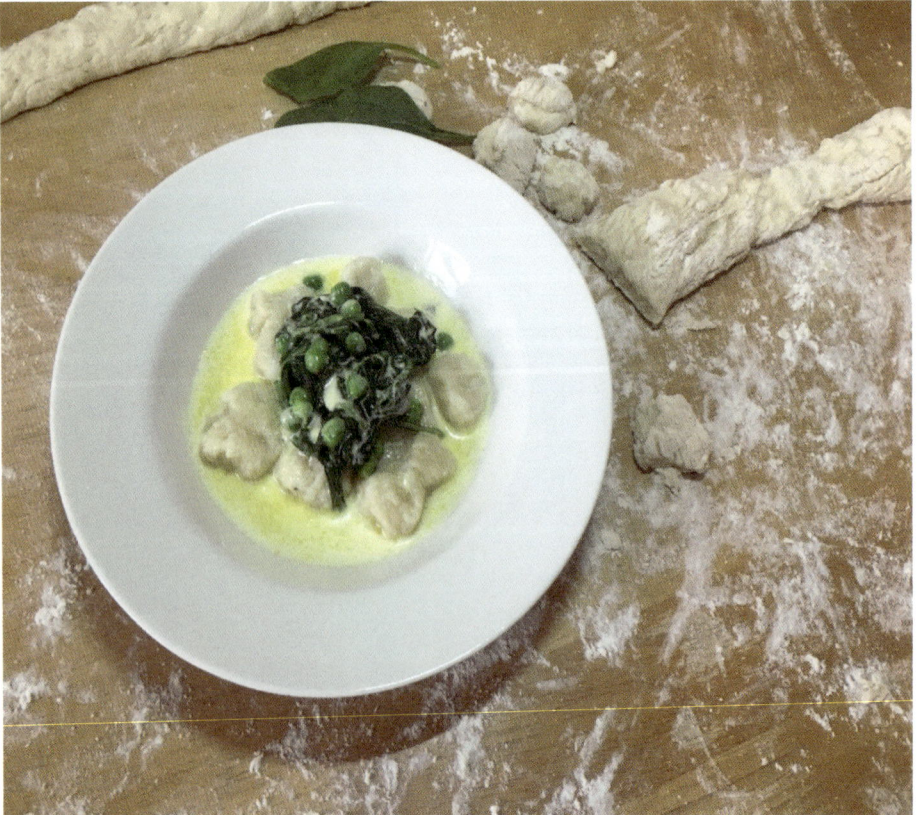

Chicken Arrabbiata

2 tbsp olive oil
2 medium onions, grated
1 bulb garlic, peeled & cloves separated
1 red chili, halved lengthways & deseeded
350ml red wine
350ml stock
600g vine tomatoes, chopped
3 tbsp tomato purée
2 tsp thyme
4 chicken breasts or 1/2 bag soy 'chicken' pieces

- Heat the oil in a large pan, fry the onion & whole garlic cloves for a few minutes, add in the two large pieces of chili (for easy removal later)
- Add the wine, allow to bubble for 1 minute then add the stock, tomatoes, tomato purée, thyme & season well with salt & pepper
- Add chicken pieces, allow to simmer 45 minutes

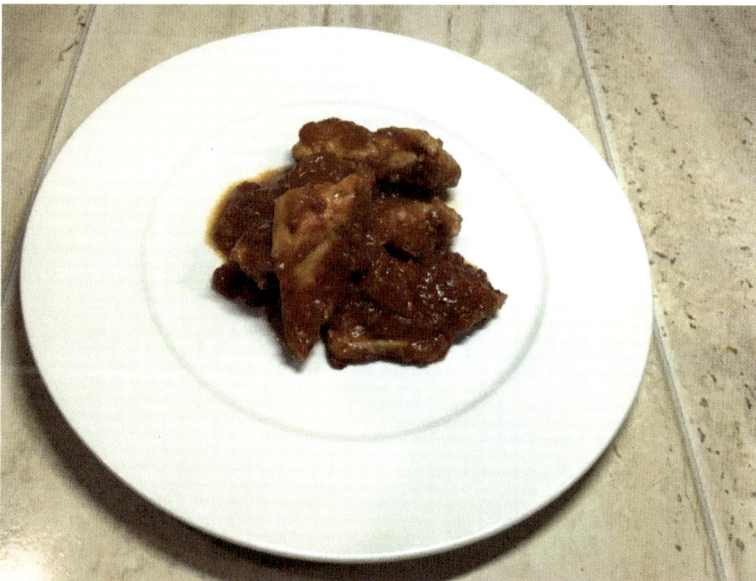

Vegetarian Comfort Food

1 packet frozen meatless sausages
3 Portobello mushrooms, chopped
1 onion, grated
1 tin chickpeas
1 tin chopped tomatoes
1/2 tsp chili flakes
1 tsp paprika
2 tbsp olive oil
1/2 tsp garlic powder
2 tbsp soy sauce
50ml red wine
2 tbsp bbq sauce
Pinch of sugar
Salt & Pepper

- Cook the sausages in the oven as per pack instructions
- In a food processor add all ingredients except for the chickpeas, combine
- Heat the oil in a large pan add the mixed ingredients, bring to a boil, then simmer
- Add the cooked sausages & chickpeas, then simmer gently for roughly 10 minutes, season well with salt & pepper.

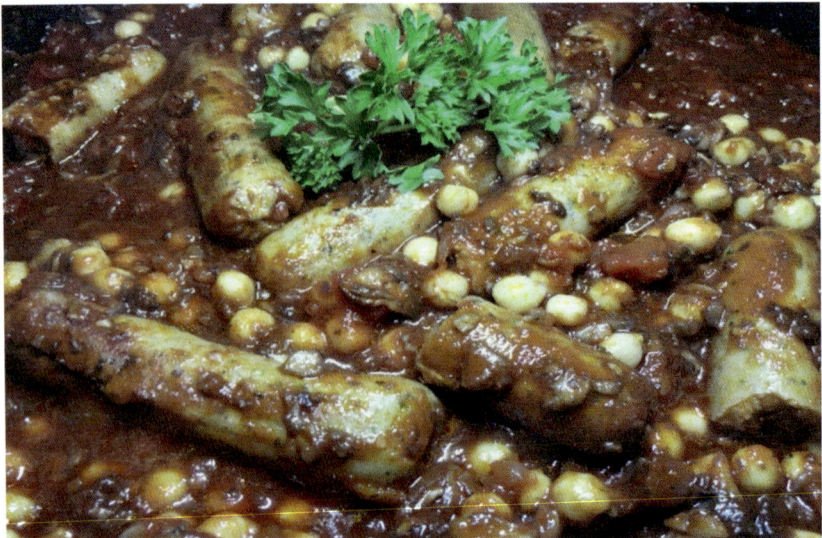

Roast Lentil Loaf

1 tbsp oil
1 medium onion, grated
3 cloves garlic, crushed
2 Portobello mushrooms, chopped
1 large carrot, grated
1 tbsp soy sauce
1 tin kidney beans, drained & rinsed
1 tin green lentils, drained & rinsed
2 tbsp mixed herbs
135g porridge oats
1 sachet nutritional yeast
1/2 tsp chili flakes
Salt & Pepper

- Preheat the oven to 190 degrees, grease and line a loaf tin with grease proof paper
- Heat the oil in a large pan add the onion & garlic & cook for 2-3 minutes add the mushroom & carrot, cook until softened add a little more oil if necessary to prevent sticking
- Add the remaining ingredients & stir well then transfer to a large mixing bowl, use a hand blender to combine & slightly purée the mixture, add a couple of tbsp water to help the mixture to combine if needed
- Transfer the mixture into the loaf tin & bake in the centre of the oven for 45-50 minutes until the outside has a crispy crust & the centre is firm
- Remove from the oven & turn out onto a serving dish, slowly & carefully remove the grease proof paper
- Serve with gravy, cranberry sauce, roast potatoes & mixed vegetables

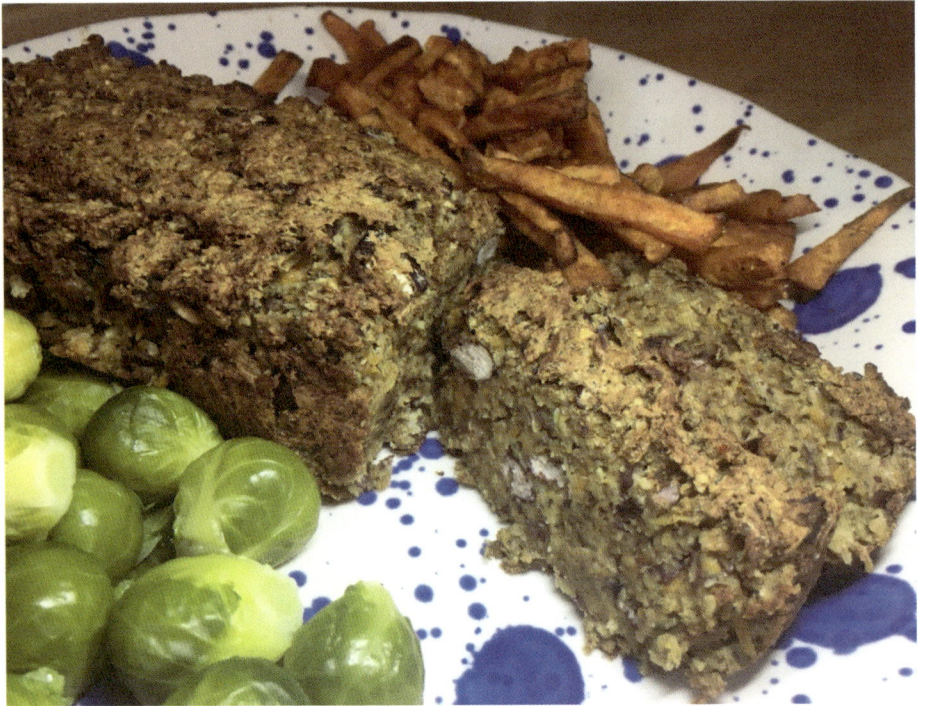

(perfect alternative to traditional Sunday Roast or Christmas dinner)

Yummy Treats

Moist Chocolate Cake / Brownies with chocolate frosting

....

150g brown sugar

300g self raising flour

1 egg
250ml fat free milk
75ml rapeseed oil
1tsp vanilla essence
6 heaped tbsp cocoa
3/4 tsp baking powder
3/4 tsp baking soda
1/2 tsp salt
100ml boiling water

Chocolate Frosting

1cup icing sugar
3 tbsp cocoa
1/2 tsp vanilla essence
2-3 tbsp hot water

- Pre-heat the oven to 180 degrees, grease & line two round cake tins or a large flat tin for brownies
- In a large bowl mix all of the dry ingredients add in the wet ones & mix well leaving the boiling water until last. Mix well with a hand blender to remove any lumps.
- At this stage you can add any extras you like such as chocolate chips, nuts or berries
- Pour the mixture in to the lined cake tins, do not fill above halfway as the liquid will rise
- This cake should remain moist, the prepared mix is quite runny, bake in the center of the oven 25-30 minutes, rotating once or twice during baking for even cooking.

Once the cake has been removed from the oven, allow to cool then turn out onto a flat surface.

Prepare the frosting by mixing all of the ingredients then drizzle the frosting over the top of the cake.

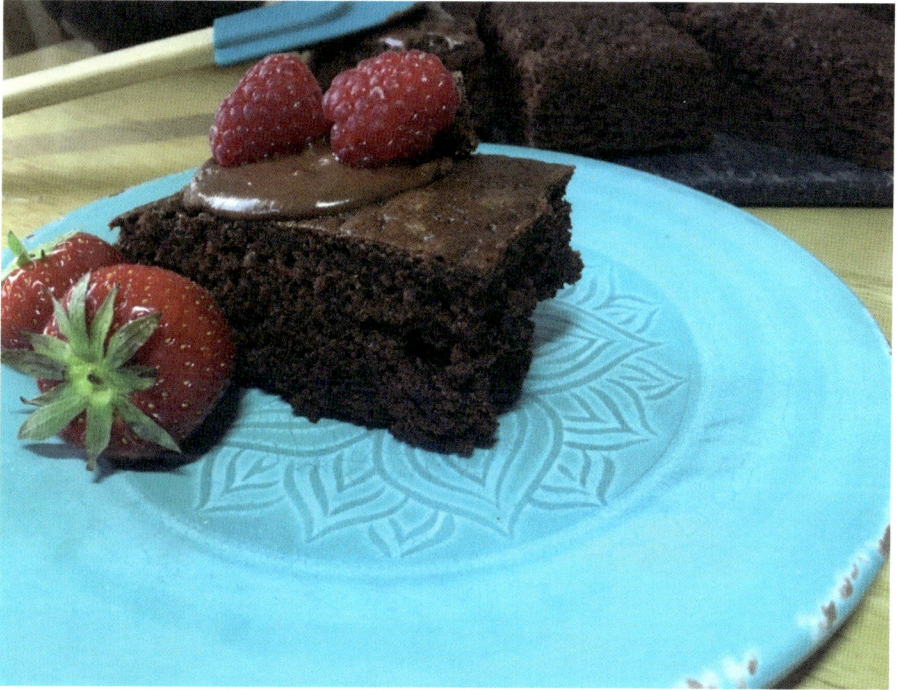

Chocolate

1 jar almond butter
5 tbsp cocoa
1. 1/4 cup reduced fat milk powder
2/3 cup powdered sugar
1/2 cup water
You can add dried cranberries to the mixture before placing it into the freezer

- Grease & line a large edged baking tray
- Sieve the powdered milk & cocoa
- Heat the water, sieve the sugar & add it to the warm water, stir until the sugar has dissolved, it will become syrupy
- Add the sieved powdered milk & cocoa, mix well
- Add the almond butter & mix well, add the cranberries if desired at this stage
- Pour the mixture into the lined edged tray & place into the freezer
- Once hardened a little use wet hands to shape into balls
- This chocolate has to be kept in the freezer as it will melt very quickly due to the low saturated fat content

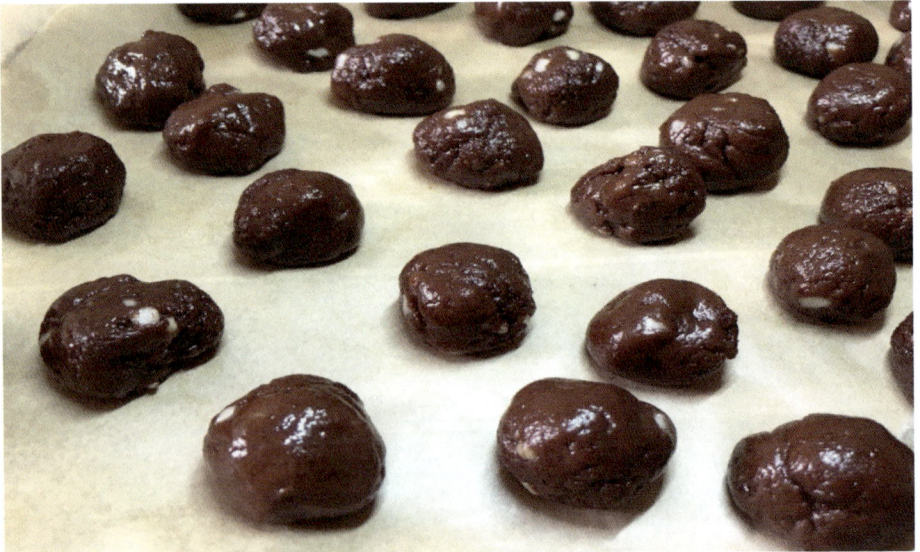

Lemon Cake

If you prefer a lighter lemon taste use less lemon juice in the mixture & use water to mix with the icing sugar instead of lemon juice.

75ml rapeseed oil
3/4 cup self raising flour
2 large eggs
2 tbsp lemon zest
Juice of 2 lemons
1/2 cup brown sugar
1/4 tsp salt
3-4 tbsp icing sugar

- Zest & juice 2 lemons, set aside

- Grease & line a loaf tin & pre-heat a fan oven to 170 degrees

- Mix the flour, sugar, salt & oil

- Beat in the eggs with 3/4 of the lemon juice

- Mix until smooth, use a hand blender if necessary

- Pour into the lined tin & bake in the center of the oven 55-60 minutes

- Remove from the oven, mix the icing sugar with the remaining lemon juice & pour the icing over the top of the cake & sprinkle with the lemon zest, allow to cool completely then remove from the tin

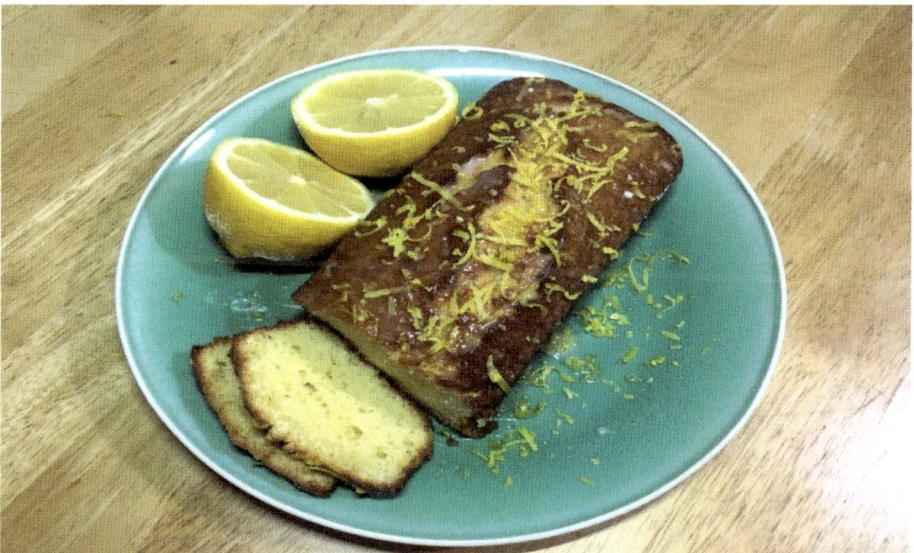

Oatmeal Cookies

Chocolate chips can be used in place of raisins.

150ml rapeseed oil
200g brown   sugar
2 egg whites
1 large egg
2 tsp vanilla essence

230g plain flour
100g porridge oats
3/4 cup raisins
1 tsp baking powder
1/4 tsp salt

- Preheat the oven to 170 degrees, line a baking tray with grease proof paper
- mix the oil & sugar add in the egg whites mix well then add in the whole egg & vanilla
- in a separate bowl combine all of the dry ingredients
- transfer the dry mixture into the wet ingredients, bit by bit, mix into a gooey dough
- drop large spoonfuls of the dough onto the lined baking sheet about 2inch apart
- use wet hands to gently press down on each cookie if necessary
- bake in the center of the oven, batch by batch (roughly 6 per batch)
- cook until firm but not too hard then remove from the oven, use a spatula to remove each cookie from the tray & allow to cool on a wire rack then drizzle with chocolate frosting if desired, as per recipe in this book.

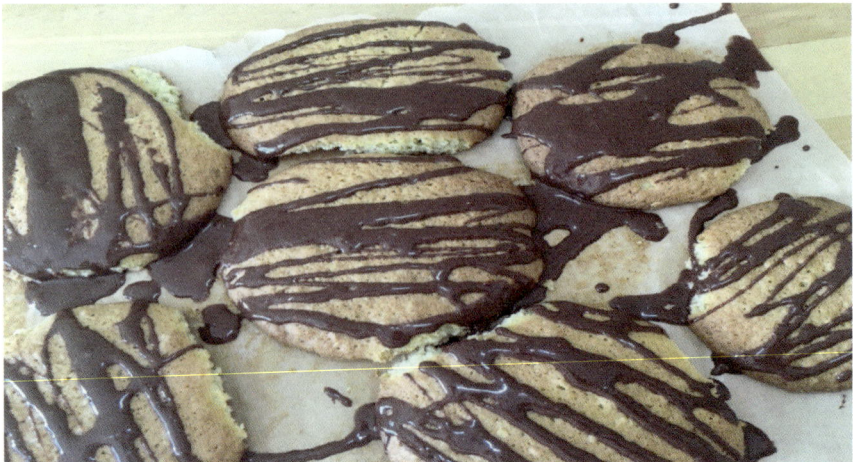

Pie Crust sweet or Savory

For savory dough i.e. quiche
100ml rapeseed oil
150ml water
400g plain flour

For sweet dough i.e. fruit pie
Add two tbsp caster sugar with the flour
Add 1tsp vanilla essence with the oil

- Mix all ingredients together
- Separate into two balls
- This dough should be rolled out between two sheets of grease proof paper
- For fruit pie, line the base of a pie dish with a sheet of the rolled dough, fill with fruit of your choice & sprinkle with sugar then place a second layer of rolled dough on top, press the edges firmly & pierce the center to allow air to escape
- Bake in the center of a pre-heated fan oven at 170 degrees for 30-35 minutes

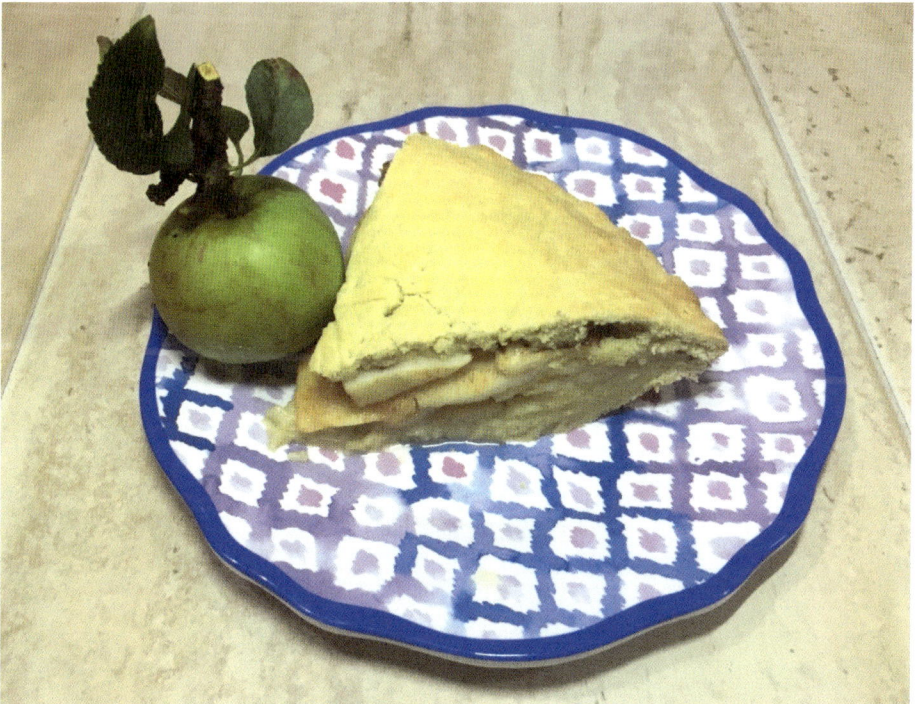

Scones

· ·

1 egg
5 tbsp rapeseed oil
100g porridge oats
150g brown sugar
270g self raising flour
1 tsp baking powder
Pinch of salt
2tbsp sultanas
175ml fat free milk
1tsp vanilla essence

- Pre-heat a fan oven to 160 degrees
- Mix oil, sugar, egg & vanilla add the dry ingredients adding the milk last, it will be a sticky breadcrumbs consistency, use your fingers to achieve this texture
- Line a muffin tin with muffin cases, drop large tablespoonfuls of the mixture into each muffin case
- Bake in the center of the oven 25-30 minutes, until golden in color
- Allow to cool then remove each scone from its muffin case

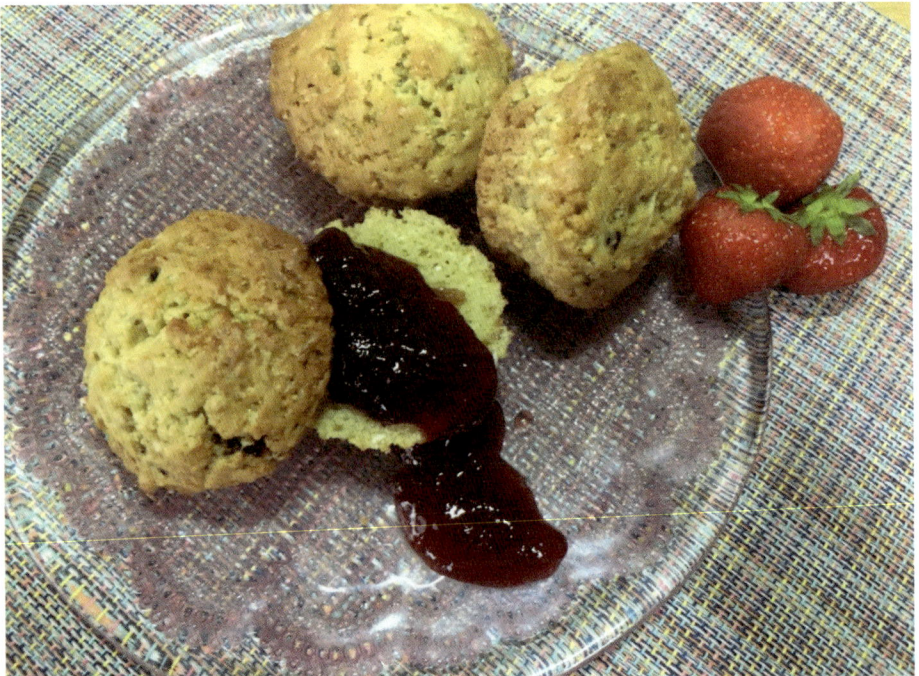

Banana Bread

3-4 ripe bananas, mashed
100ml rapeseed oil
150g brown sugar
1tsp vanilla essence
1tsp baking powder
270g self raising flour
Pinch of salt
Runny honey to drizzle

- Grease & line a loaf tin, pre-heat the oven to 150 degrees

- Mix the bananas & oil, add in the egg, sugar & vanilla

- Mix in the flour, salt & baking powder

- Pour the mixture into the lined loaf tin

- Bake in the center of the oven until risen & a wooden skewer inserted into the middle comes out clean, 55-60 minutes

- Once removed from the oven drizzle honey over the top & leave to cool in the tin

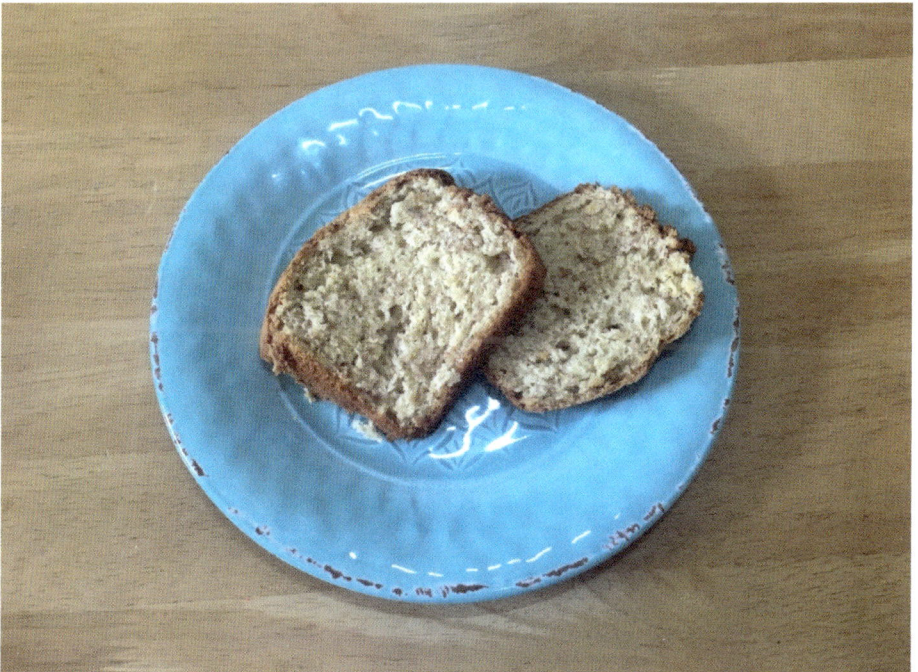

Marshmallow Rice Krispie Treats

2-3 tbsp grapeseed oil

300g bag white or pink marshmallows

300g rice krispies

- Line a deep dish with grease proof paper

- In a large pot heat the oil add the marshmallows, stirring continuously until they melt into a thick liquid, keep them on a low temperature being careful not to burn

- Continue to stir & add the rice krispies

- Once rice krispies have been coated transfer the sticky mess into the dish

- Use wet hands to flatten the mixture to fill the dish

- Leave to cool, then turn out & cut into shapes.

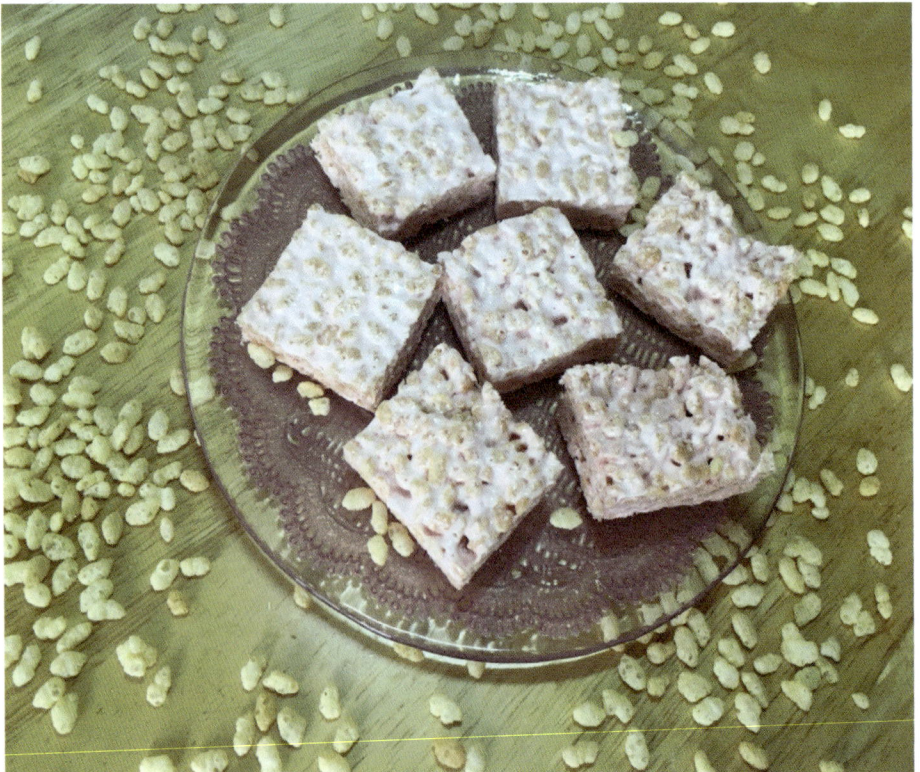

French Toast

Sliced brioche bread or sliced bread of your choice
2 large eggs
50ml non fat milk
Pinch of salt
1-2 tsp grapeseed oil

- In a flat bowl whisk together the eggs, milk & salt
- Heat the oil in a pan until hot but not smoking
- Quickly dip each side of 1 slice of bread into the egg mixture to fully coat the bread with the mixture, do not allow to soak
- Place the coated bread onto the hot pan & cook on both sides 30 seconds to a minute per side, being careful not to burn
- Repeat until the mixture is finished, this mixture will make roughly 4 slices
- Serve drizzled with maple syrup, fresh berries or simply plain

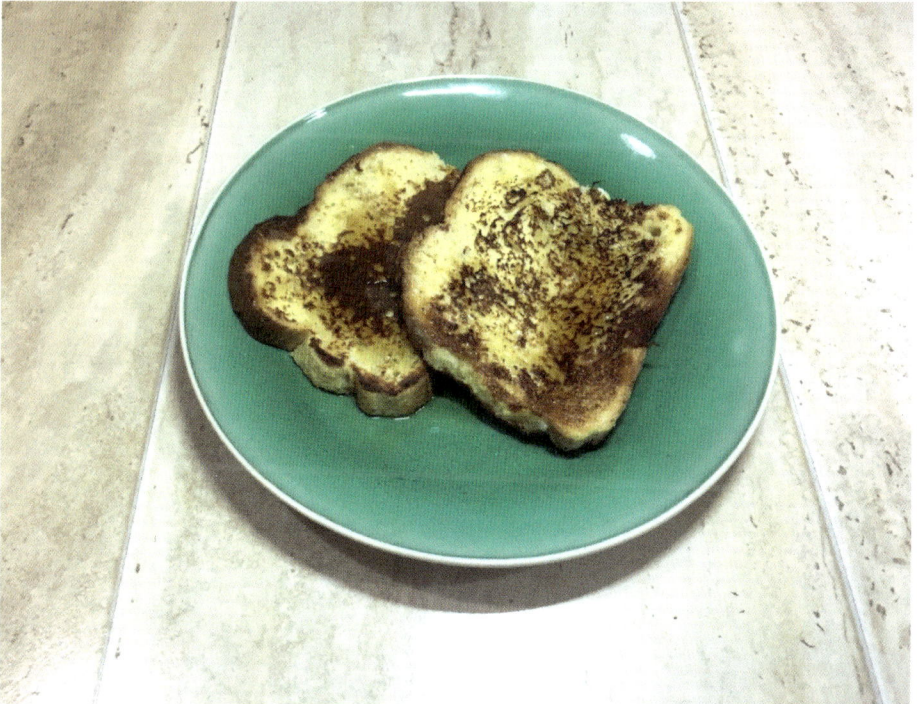

Energy Balls

• •

1 cup pitted dates
1 cup raw cashew nuts
2 tsp vanilla essence
1/2 tsp Himalayan pink salt
85g vegan dark chocolate
Wooden toothpicks

- In a food processor blend the dates, cashews, vanilla & salt
- The mixture will be a sticky breadcrumbs consistency, spoon the mixture out onto a large sheet of grease proof paper then using your hands take small handfuls & press the mixture together to make small bite sized balls
- Insert a toothpick into the centre of each one
- In a small pot heat some water & place a large bowl on top, break the chocolate into small pieces & melt them in the bowl
- Once the chocolate has melted dip each ball to coat it fully in the chocolate
- Then stand on a sheet of greaseproof paper to dry

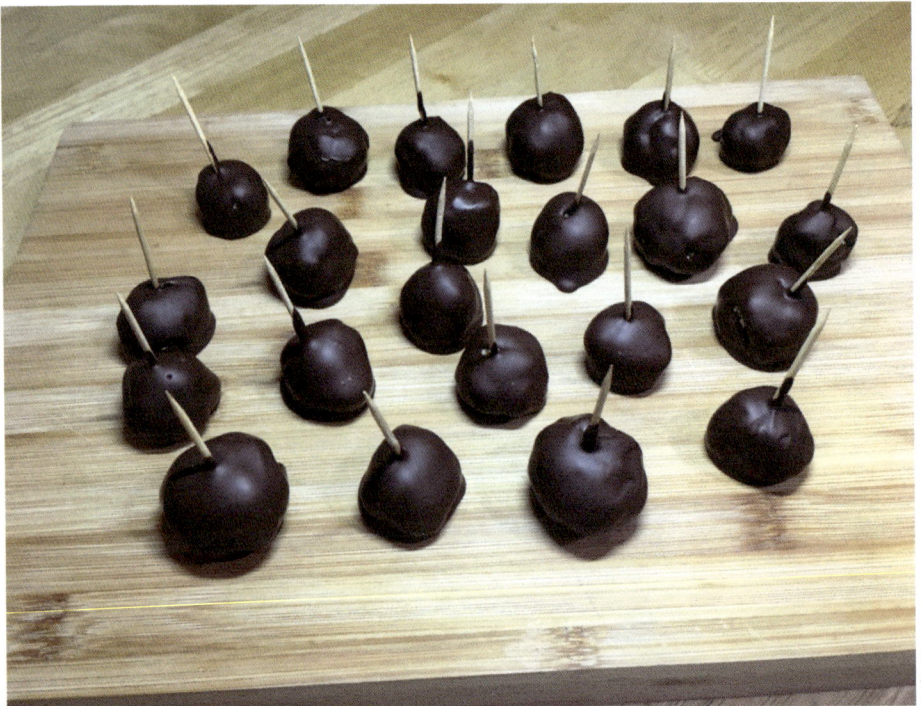

Vegan Cinnamon Swirls

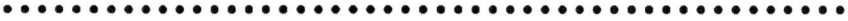

240ml almond milk
100ml rapeseed oil
410g self raising flour + extra for kneading
1 sachet yeast
1/4 tsp salt
1.5 tsp ground cinnamon
1tbsp brown sugar + extra for topping

Frosting
110g icing sugar
1-2 tbsp almond milk
1tsp vanilla essence

- Heat the almond milk in a large pot, once warm add the oil, bring to 33 - 39 degrees (not above or below or the yeast won't activate)
- Transfer the liquid to a large mixing bowl add the sugar & salt, stir then sprinkle the yeast on top, stir gently then leave for 10 minutes
- Add the flour little by little, combining with each flour addition until you achieve sticky dough
- Turn out onto a floured surface & knead for a minute or so, clean the mixing bowl then brush lightly with oil. Place the dough into the oiled bowl, cover with cling film & leave it in a warm place to rise for about an hour
- Once the dough has risen, turn out once again onto a floured surface & roll out into a large rectangle & brush lightly with oil, mix the cinnamon & sugar then sprinkle it generously onto the dough, be sure to cover it completely, add more cinnamon & sugar if necessary
- At the long side of the dough rectangle roll the dough into a long sausage shape then use a sharp knife to slice it into each cinnamon swirl
- Lightly oil a large baking dish & place each cinnamon swirl into the dish, at this stage the swirls can be covered with cling film & left over night to cook fresh in the morning or you can bake them straight away
- Preheat the oven to 180 degrees & bake the cinnamon swirls in the centre of the oven for 25-30 minutes
- Combine the frosting ingredients, then pour in straight lines over the swirls

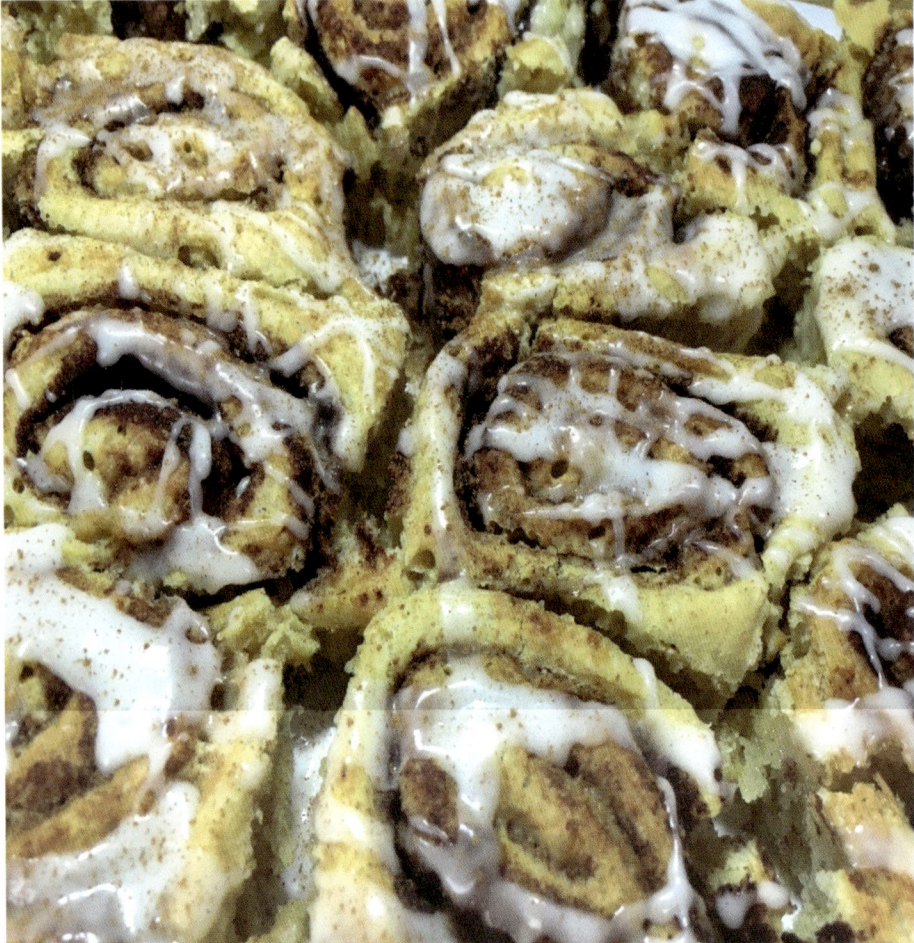

28305159R00031

Printed in Great Britain
by Amazon